Dental Pain Relief
(Using Nutrition & Sleeping Position)
&
Back Pain Relief
(Using Nutrition only)

No more toothaches; no more gum pains
No more visits or less visits to dental offices

No more lower back pains; no more waist pains; no more spinal manipulations; no more or less visits to chiropractic offices

A. A. FREMPONG

Dental Pain Relief & Back Pain Relief

Copyright © 2018 by A. A. Frempong

Published by Yellowtextbooks.com. N.Y. All Rights Reserved.
No part of this book may be reproduced in any form
without written permission from the publisher.

ISBN 978-1-946485-70-0

Printed in the United States of America

In Memory of My Parents

Mom:
She was a devoted mother, sharing, kind, kinder to strangers and generous to a fault. She never cursed, she never hated; she never cheated, and she never envied. She never lied, and she never got angry. Once, she nursed an almost dying stranger renting a room in her house back to good health to the extent that the relatives of this renter later travelled one hundred miles just to thank mom. She was always peaceloving and forever forgiving. An angel once lived on this earth to serve others.

Dad:
A great dad, kind, generous and forgiving. He emphasized and was an example of both formal education and self-education. A veterinarian, a bacteriologist, an Associate of the Institute of Medical Laboratory Technology (UK), a Fellow of the Royal Society of Health (UK); an incorruptible civil servant; his book on ticks has always inspired me to write whenever the need arises.

Preface

I never thought of becoming the messenger to discover cures for dental pains (toothache, gum pains) and back pains (lower, waist, middle, upper), and similar pains; and I never thought of writing a book on health care, having published the most user-friendly mathematics titles (from arithmetic to Calculus), until for the first time, I had some toothache, and I was able to relieve the pain within a few days by proper positioning of my body when sleeping. I cannot keep such a miraculous and healthy experience to myself, but share it.

Discovery of procedures for dental pain relief

I got up from bed one morning and experienced a toothache for the first time. I tried to find a reason why I had the toothache, and tried to reason that it was due to lack of sunshine. I also thought that it was due to an infection, and therefore, I chewed some ginger, but the pain got worse. I discontinued the ginger treatment. For the next few days, I went out to get some sunshine and it seemed that exposure to sunlight had helped to reduce the pain. Some days later, according to the weather forecast, there would not be any sunshine for the next three days. At night, without exposure to sunlight during the day, I went to sleep, and when I woke up the next morning, the toothache had subsided, even without exposure to sunlight the day before. I reflected and came to the conclusion that the pain reduction was due to my sleeping on my stomach during sleep, the night before. From that day on, I repeated sleeping on my stomach for the next two days without exposure to sunlight during the day, but the pain subsided. From those days on, I made sure that I slept on my stomach for some hours when sleeping. Without seeking any medical attention, the toothache vanished, and also my gums felt better. It has been five years now, since I last felt any dental pain or discomfort. I wondered why I had not heard or read that sleeping on one's stomach improves one's dental health. From the above experience, I concluded that the two main requirements that must be satisfied simultaneously, in order to relieve dental pain (toothache, gum pain, etc.) and maintain good dental health are proper nutrition and the proper positioning of the human body (i.e., sleeping on one's stomach, for some hours) when sleeping.

Discovery of procedures for back pain relief

About six years before the toothache experience, I had some lower back pain, and was able to relieve the pain within five to seven days by adding broccoli to my diet, twice a day for the first five days. I continued to eat the broccoli, but only once a day for ten years. After ten years, I stopped eating the broccoli or did not eat it very often, but the pain did not return. Some months later, I drank some herbal tea for sleeping, and after about an hour, I felt uncomfortable, and the next morning, I felt a sharp lower back pain. Immediately, I knew what to do (applying my experience ten years before). I ate the broccoli twice a day, and within five days, the pain had vanished. I therefore concluded that I had really found a cure for back pain (upper back, middle back, waist or lower back). When I went online to the web, I realized that my experience can help over 30 million Americans and millions of people worldwide, and prevent disabilities worldwide, provided people become aware of the suggestions in this book.

Other books by the author: Integrated Arithmetic; Elementary Algebra; Intermediate Algebra, Elementary Mathematics; Intermediate Mathematics; Elementary & Intermediate Mathematics (combined); College Algebra; College Trigonometry; College Algebra & Trigonometry, Calculus 1 & 2 and Final Exam Review titles and Power of Ratios.

Contents

Page

CHAPTER A 1
Dental Pain Relief 1
Summary 1
Food Preparation Instructions 2
Breakfast 2
Lunch 4
Dinner 5
Discussion and Conclusion 7

CHAPTER B 8
Back Pain Relief 8
Summary 8
Food Preparation Instructions 9
Breakfast 9
Lunch 11
Dinner 12
Discussion and Conclusion 14

CHAPTER A
Dental Pain Relief
Using Nutrition & Sleeping Position
Summary

This chapter covers procedures for relieving dental pain using nutrition and the proper positioning of the human body when sleeping. The relief procedures are based on the author's personal experience during the past five years. The nutritional requirements are eggs, tomato, onion. celery and **broccoli**. For breakfast, one will prepare a fried **egg-tomato-onion combination** and a cup of an 8-minute boiled broccoli. The procedures involved are important to the dental pain relief as well as one's health. For lunch, one will prepare an appetizing soup using chicken, tomato, onion, baby carrots, celery and sardines in oil or in tomato sauce. For dinner, one will boil some rice and eat this with the 1/4 of the egg-tomato-onion combination left-over from the breakfast preparation. One can add some green vegetables to the dinner meal. The main requirements are the ingredients, the food preparation method, and the proper positioning of the human body when sleeping. It is important that after the pain relief, one continues with the diet and the body positioning when sleeping, but reduces the frequency of the **broccoli** consumption to three or four times a week. Note that one is eating food and not taking medicine; and when it comes to food, one will continue to eat for the rest of one's life. After searching the web, the author was surprised that no remedy for dental pain relief mentioned the positioning of the human body when sleeping.

Solution to Dental Pain Problems

The solution consists of a nutritious breakfast with broccoli, a nutritious lunch, a nutritious dinner and the proper positioning of the human body when sleeping. Note that from my experience, the proper positioning of the body during sleep is critical to a good dental health, because when I had the toothache, I did not change my diet. The only change was the proper positioning of my body during sleep. The beauty in this remedy nutrition and body positioning is that people are used to them, except the awareness, and perhaps, the frequency requirements of the body positioning. Below, I present the nutritional requirements based on what I had been eating and still eating. I cannot eliminate any of the ingredients.

Food Preparation Instructions
Breakfast, Lunch & Dinner

Breakfast

Ingredients
1. 2 eggs (brown eggs preferred), fresh tomato, fresh onion, salt, sardines in oil
2. Unsalted crackers (e.g., unsalted Crich or Sophia crackers, a product of Italy) instead of bread.
3. Oats (such as Quaker Oats), or corn flour or corn meal for preparing porridge.
4. Broccoli florets.

> **Step 1**: At time $t = 0$, some cooking vegetable oil (e.g. Mazola corn oil) is poured into a frying pan on a stove with very low flame. Cut pieces of onion, and tomato are placed in the frying pan containing the oil and some salt (very small amount) is sprinkled over the contents of the frying pan. Obtain a piece of the sardine in oil, break it into pieces and sprinkle the pieces into the contents of the frying pan. Cover the contents and let them fry for about **5** minutes. Beat-up two fresh eggs in a saucepan to mix the yellow and white parts of the eggs. Remove the cover and pour the egg mixture into to the contents and stir thoroughly. Cover the contents, and fry for another **5** minutes. Remove the cover and stir the contents to break-up the contents. Cover them and let the contents fry for another 3 minutes; and turn off the fire. Remove and place the contents on a plate and drain off the oil in the contents by tilting the plate.

Step 2: Prepare the oats or corn porridge. Add sugar and milk. (Learn how to prepare porridge)

Step 3: Boil about a cup of broccoli for 8 minutes.
Boil the broccoli for about 8 minutes, and importantly, do not over-boil (the color of the broccoli should still be green when you stop boiling. If the color is not green (color becomes somewhat gray, do not eat the broccoli; but boil a new a cup of broccoli. When the broccoli in a cooking utensil is placed on a fire, it takes about 4-5 minutes before the water begins to "boil" ; and after another 4 minutes; turn off the fire and immediately drain the water off the broccoli. I inadvertently consumed over-boiled broccoli for a number of days and experienced a sharp lower back pain.

Step 4: **For breakfast**, eat the following: about three fourths of the contents from Step 1; (save the remaining one fourth for dinner); the boiled broccoli with some tomato ketch-up on it, the crackers and the porridge.
 Do not eat butter, margarine or cheese of any brand. Your cholesterol level will be safe because of the tomato-onion combination with the eggs.

Eating the breakfast:

Start with a piece of the crackers into the mouth, then some egg-tomato-onion combination, start chewing and add a piece of the broccoli, continue chewing, then add some porridge; and repeat the process. Avoid eating for instance all the broccoli, then all the porridge. Mix up the ingredients into your stomach.

Water after every meal
 Cut an orange into two halves and eat one half with a cup of water (or you may drink a cup of orange juice).

Lunch

Preparation of an Appetizing Ashanti Light Soup

Ingredients:
1. Three chicken legs (drumsticks).
2. One bulb of fresh onion.
3. One medium "bulb" of fresh tomato.
4. Salt (sprinkle conservatively on the chicken).
   To gauge the amount of salt, just sprinkle on the tops of two of the chicken legs only.
   You can add more salt after cooking.
   Note that too much salt may be irreversible.
5. Sardines in tomato sauce or in oil.
6. Fresh baby carrots (about 8, 1-inch pieces).
7. Celery.
8. A mixture of green beans, peas, and sweet corn

Method

Step 1: At time t = 0: Three chicken legs, onion, carrots, celery, a mixture of green beans, peas, and sweet corn **and** some salt are placed in a cooking utensil. **Do not add any water at this time.** The contents are heated (for about 15 minutes using very low flame, stirring the contents every two minutes. The contents will turn gray with a pleasant onion odor. The first 15 minutes are critical; so watch the contents very carefully, otherwise, they would burn.

Step 2: At time, t = 15 minutes, freshly cut tomato are added to the contents (place the tomato pieces near the walls of the cooking utensil), and boiled for about 15 more minutes. Using a spoon, press the tomatoes against the walls of the cooking utensil to flatten and grind them. You may grind the fresh tomato and just add the juice.

Step 3: At time t =30 minutes, ground fresh tomato or tomato paste, sardines in tomato sauce, are added; followed by 3 to 4 cups of water, "Turn up the flame" now. The contents are boiled for another 50-60 minutes.

Step 4: At time, t = 90 minutes, turn off the fire, and an appetizing soup would be ready. You may also add 10 extra minutes in Step 4 if you want to thicken the soup.

Extra: (In Step 1, you may include fresh crabs (regular crabs). The soup may be served with cocoyam, yam, green plantains, mashed potato, boiled potatoes; and fufu (prepared from mashed potato and potato starch) etc.

Note above that you may increase or decrease the duration of the boiling for each step by experimentation and experience.

Dinner

Boil some rice, and eat it with some vegetables and the 1/4 of the egg-tomato-onion combination left-over from the breakfast preparation. You may also add some unsalted crackers, and a small piece of the chicken left-over from the lunch soup to the rice.

Water after every meal
Cut an orange into two halves and eat one half with a cup of water (or you may drink a cup of orange juice).

Exercising
When you get up in the morning, you may exercise on a one-wheel stationary cycle. Do not sit on the cycle seat. Place your right foot on the left pedal and pedal, followed by placing your left foot on the right pedal and pedaling. Also swing simultaneously your two hands up and down your sides up to your head. Also you may try shadow boxing using open hands as well as fisted hands. You may swing simultaneously, both of your hands from left to right in front of you. Walk outside home everyday for 30 minutes, and if possible, face the sun while walking.

Going to bed and body positioning when sleeping

Sleep on a flat wooden bed with lightweight firm polyurethane foam mattress. Your bed's height should be such that when you sit on the edge of the bed, your feet touch the floor flatly. I took measurements of my desired bed, went to a lumber yard, and the parts (wooden parts) of the bed were cut for me. I also went to where lightweight polyurethane foam mattresses are cut to size for customers. Using a hammer and nails, I put the parts together to form my desired bed. The bed should be firm but comfortable. When you go to bed, sleep on your stomach. **Note** that sleeping on the stomach implies that you sleep for some hours on your stomach and for some hours on your back. When you sleep on your stomach, you turn your head a little bit to the left or to the right on the pillow to ease breathing. If a pain is on the left side of the mouth, turn your head to the right on the pillow; but if the pain is on the right side of the mouth, turn your head to the left on the pillow. That is put pressure on the side with pain.

After the pain relief
After the pain has completely vanished, continue with your new diet and the sleeping on the stomach position. You may try eating broccoli only 3 or 4 times a week. Learn from your experience. You are the best doctor for you. Share your experience with the people you meet when possible.

If possible, avoid eating food prepared outside home in order to keep track of what goes into your stomach.

Sunshine:
Get some sunshine as often as possible;
Also, no alcohol (do not listen to people using words like "moderation".

Discussion and Conclusion

About the eggs

I had been eating 2 eggs a day for many years and when I had a clinical lab examination, the clinical lab report said that my cholesterol level was satisfactory. I was surprised that the cholesterol level was normal after eating two eggs a day for many years. I had to come up with reasons why the cholesterol level was normal and not high. One reason I came up with is that the eggs were mixed with onions and tomato when fried and also I had heard that onion and tomato reduce the cholesterol level in blood. Recently on television, I heard that the cholesterol in the blood is not due to eggs. Therefore, one should not be concerned with eating eggs, the best source of protein. However, I suggest that one should **not** eat margarine, butter or cheese of any kind (to avoid raising the level of triglycerides in blood); and off course, **no alcohol.** After a few months, you may ask a doctor for a clinical lab test to determine your blood cholesterol level. Always, remember that experience is the best teacher; and one can make modifications with time and experience. After searching the web, I was surprised that no remedy for the relief of dental pains mentioned or emphasized body positioning when sleeping. Finally, when possible and convenient, share your experience with others in need.

Possible reasons why sleeping on the stomach helps to reduce dental pain

When one sleeps on the stomach, one presses the contents of the mouth (teeth, tongue and gums etc.) together, helping the blood cells do their work. The blood flowing into this location may stay a little bit longer than otherwise. Also, the gravitational effect on the dental parts is different from sleeping on one's back. Pressing the contents of the mouth together could be similar to bandaging a sore on the skin for healing.

Extra: The best position for a baby in the mother's womb just before birth is the baby's head facing down and facing the mother's back. This position is called the "occipito-anterior" position. So, quite naturally, after birth, this position should be continued and approximated by sleeping on the stomach for some hours when sleeping, since such a position would be continuing the baby's position just before birth. If a baby is born prematurely, perhaps, this position should be approximated and included in the baby's positioning when sleeping, to facilitate completion of development. A special equipment could be built to facilitate this sleeping position, with provision to facilitate breathing. It is suggested that to reduce disorders such as cleft lips and palates, as soon as possible, during pregnancy, babies should be encouraged to move into or be moved into the "occipito-anterior" position. If this position is not detrimental to the baby's development early in the pregnancy, then this should be the baby's position as soon as possible.

It is predicted that sleeping on the stomach also affects, positively, the senses of vision, hearing, taste, smell and touch. Thus, eating well and sleeping on the stomach could help solve problems of vision, hearing, taste, smell, and touch.

Always, remember that you are the best doctor for you.

CHAPTER B
Back Pain Relief Using Nutrition
Summary

This chapter covers procedures for relieving back pain and similar pains using nutrition. The relief procedures are based on the author's personal experience during the past ten years. The main ingredients are eggs, **broccoli**, tomato, and onion. For breakfast, one will prepare a fried **egg-tomato-onion combination** and a cup of an 8-minute boiled broccoli. The procedure used in the food preparation is important to the pain relief as well as one's health. For lunch, one will prepare an appetizing soup using chicken, tomato, onion, baby carrots, celery and sardines in oil or in tomato sauce. For dinner, one will boil some rice and also boil a cup of broccoli and eat this with the 1/4 of the egg-tomato-onion combination left-over from the breakfast preparation. The main requirements are the ingredients, the preparation method, how many times a day the **broccoli** is eaten, and for how many days continuously it is eaten. It is important that after the pain relief, one continues with the diet; but reduces the frequency of the **broccoli** consumption to once a day (or half a cup at breakfast and half a cup at dinner). Note that one is eating food and not taking medicine; and when it comes to food, one will continue to eat for the rest of one's life. The solution for the back pain problem is a needed diet and not medication. A nutritious breakfast with broccoli, a nutritious lunch, and a nutritious dinner with **broccoli** will alleviate the pains. The beauty in this remedy nutrition is that people are used to it, except the frequency, and perhaps, the food preparation requirements. After searching the web, the author was surprised that no remedy for the pain relief emphasized nutrition.

Seniors Walking With Canes

One of the reasons some seniors walk with canes is nutritional deficiency and not old age. The solution is a needed diet and not medication. A nutritious breakfast with broccoli, a nutritious lunch, and a nutritious dinner with broccoli will alleviate the pains involved.

Food Preparation Instructions
Breakfast

Ingredients

1. 2 eggs (brown eggs preferred), fresh tomato, fresh onion, salt, sardines in oil.
2. Unsalted crackers (e.g., unsalted Crich or Sophia crackers, a product of Italy) instead of bread.
3. Oats (such as Quaker Oats), or corn flour or corn meal for preparing porridge.
4. Broccoli florets.

Step 1: At time $t = 0$, some cooking vegetable oil (e.g. Mazola corn oil) is poured into a frying pan on a stove with very low flame. Cut pieces of onion, and tomato are placed in the frying pan containing the oil and some salt (very small amount) is sprinkled over the contents of the frying pan. Obtain a piece of the sardine in oil, break it into pieces and sprinkle the pieces into the contents of the frying pan. Cover the contents and let them fry for about **5** minutes. Beat-up two fresh eggs in a saucepan to mix the yellow and white parts of the eggs. Remove the cover and pour the egg mixture into to the contents and stir thoroughly. Cover the contents, and fry for another **5** minutes. Remove the cover and stir the contents to break-up the contents. Cover them and let the contents fry for another 3 minutes; and turn off the fire. Remove and place the contents on a plate and drain off the oil in the contents by tilting the plate.

Step 2: Prepare the oats or corn porridge. Add sugar and milk. (Learn how to prepare porridge)

Step 3: Boil about a cup of broccoli for 8 minutes.
Boil the broccoli for about 8 minutes, and importantly, do not over-boil (the color of the broccoli should still be green when you stop boiling. If the color is not green (color becomes somewhat gray, do not eat the broccoli; but boil a new a cup of broccoli. When the broccoli in a cooking utensil is placed on a fire, it takes about 4-5 minutes before the water begins to "boil" ; and after another 4 minutes; turn off the fire and immediately drain the water off the broccoli. I inadvertently consumed over-boiled broccoli for a number of days and experienced a sharp lower back pain.

Step 4: **For breakfast,** eat the following: about three fourths of the contents from Step 1; (save the remaining one fourth for dinner); the boiled broccoli with some tomato ketch-up on it, the crackers and the porridge.

Do not eat butter, margarine or cheese of any brand. Your cholesterol level will be safe because of the tomato-onion combination with the eggs.

Eating the breakfast:

Start with a piece of the crackers into the mouth, then some egg-tomato-onion combination, start chewing and add a piece of the broccoli, continue chewing, then add some porridge; and repeat the process. Avoid eating for instance all the broccoli, then all the porridge. Mix up the ingredients into your stomach.

Water after every meal
Cut an orange into two halves and eat one half with a cup of water (or you may drink a cup of orange juice).

Lunch

Preparation of an Appetizing Ashanti Light Soup

Ingredients:
1. Three chicken legs (drumsticks).
2. One bulb of fresh onion.
3. One medium "bulb" of fresh tomato.
4. Salt (sprinkle conservatively on the chicken).
   To gauge the amount of salt, just sprinkle on the tops of two of the chicken legs only. You can add more salt after cooking. Note that too much salt may be irreversible.
5. Sardines in tomato sauce or in oil.
6. Fresh baby carrots (about 8, 1-inch pieces).
7. Celery.
8. A mixture of green beans, peas, and sweet corn

Method

Step 1: At time $t = 0$: Three chicken legs, onion, carrots, celery, a mixture of green beans, peas, and sweet corn **and** some salt are placed in a cooking utensil. **Do not add any water at this time.** The contents are heated (for about 15 minutes using very low flame, stirring the contents every two minutes. The contents will turn gray with a pleasant onion odor. The first 15 minutes are critical; so watch the contents very carefully, otherwise, they would burn.

Step 2: At time, $t = 15$ minutes, freshly cut tomato are added to the contents (place the tomato pieces near the walls of the cooking utensil), and boiled for about 15 more minutes. Using a spoon, press the tomatoes against the walls of the cooking utensil to flatten and grind them. You may grind the fresh tomato and just add the juice.

Step 3: At time t = 30 minutes, ground fresh tomato or tomato paste, sardines in tomato sauce, are added; followed by 3 to 4 cups of water, "Turn up the flame" now. The contents are boiled for another 50-60 minutes.

Step 4: At time, t = 90 minutes, turn off the fire, and an appetizing soup would be ready. You may also add 10 extra minutes in Step 4 if you want to thicken the soup.

Extra: (In Step 1, you may include fresh crabs (regular crabs). The soup may be served with cocoyam, yam, green plantains, mashed potato, boiled potatoes; and fufu (prepared from mashed potato and potato starch) etc.

Note above that you may increase or decrease the duration of the boiling for each step by experimentation and experience.

Dinner

Boil some rice or cocoyam or something similar; boil a cup of broccoli (florets) and eat the rice (cocoyam), the broccoli (with tomato ketch-up on) with the 1/4 of the egg-tomato-onion combination left-over from the breakfast preparation. You may also add a small piece of the chicken left-over from the lunch soup to the rice. Eat the rice and **broccoli** with unsalted crackers.

A note about eating broccoli

When the back pain is felt, it is critical that you eat the **broccoli** twice a day (that is, with breakfast and with dinner), for five consecutive days until the pain vanishes. Afterwards, eat the broccoli once a day, perhaps with dinner..

Water after every meal

Cut an orange into two halves and eat one half with a cup of water (or you may drink a cup of orange juice).

Fruits:

Eat some kiwifruit.

Exercising

When you get up in the morning, you may exercise on one-wheel stationary cycle. Do not sit on the cycle seat, Place your right foot on the left pedal and pedal, followed by placing your left foot on the right pedal and pedaling. Also swing simultaneously your two hands up and down your sides up to your head. Also you may try shadow boxing using open hands as well as fisted hands. You may swing simultaneously, both of your hands from left to right in front of you. Walk outside home everyday for 30 minutes, and if possible, face the sun while walking.

After the pain relief

After the pain has completely vanished, continue with your new diet, but for the broccoli, eat it once a day; and any time the pains come back, eat the broccoli twice a day for about 3-4 days (or until the pain vanishes) and then switch the broccoli consumption to once a day. with time, you may try eating broccoli only 3 or 4 times a week. Learn from experience. You are the best doctor for you. Share your experience with the people you meet when possible.

Bed

Sleep on a flat wooden bed with lightweight firm polyurethane foam mattress. Your bed's height should be such that when you sit on the edge of the bed, your feet touch the floor flatly. I took measurements of my desired bed, went to a lumber yard, and the parts (wooden parts) of the bed were cut for me. I also went to where lightweight polyurethane foam mattresses are cut to size for customers. Using a hammer and nails, I put the parts together to form my desired bed. The bed should be firm but comfortable.

Also, no alcohol (do not listen to people using words like "moderation").

Discussion and Conclusion

About the eggs
I had been eating 2 eggs a day for many years and when I had a clinical lab examination, the clinical lab report said that my cholesterol level was satisfactory. I was surprised that the cholesterol level was normal after eating two eggs a day for many years. I had to come up with reasons why the cholesterol level was normal and not high. One reason I came up with is that the eggs were mixed with onions and tomato when fried and also I had heard that onion and tomato reduce the cholesterol level in blood. Recently on television, I heard that the cholesterol in the blood is not due to eggs. Therefore, one should not be concerned with eating eggs, the best source of protein. However, I suggest that one should **not** eat margarine, butter or cheese of any kind (to avoid raising the level of triglycerides in blood); and off course, **no alcohol.** After a few months, you may ask a doctor for a clinical lab test to determine your blood cholesterol level. Always, remember that experience is the best teacher; and one can make modifications with time and experience. After searching the web, I was surprised that no remedy for the relief of back pains mentioned or emphasized eating broccoli twice a day for about 3-5 days, when there is back pain,, and then switching to eating broccoli once a day after the pain relief. Finally, when possible, and convenient, share your experience with others in need.

Note; Broccoli boiling time
When the broccoli in a cooking utensil is placed on a fire, it takes about 4-5 minutes before the water begins to "boil" ; and after another 4 minutes; turn off the fire and immediately drain the water off the broccoli.

If broccoli is not over-boiled, with tomato ketchup on, it is appetizing. When it is overboiled, it is not appetizing, and it is bad for consumption.

Extra broccoli benefit
Broccoli has positive effects on the respiratory system. By eating broccoli for the past ten years, I have not had catarrh or common cold..

Watching what you eat or drink or what you used to eat or drink
If you suddenly have a back pain, not from any physical exertion, always try to reflect on what you have recently eaten (or drunk) or what you used to eat (or drink) and have stopped eating (or drinking).

If you give your body the nutrients it needs, it will perform pleasant miracles.

Always, remember that you are the best doctor for you.

INDEX

A
About the eggs 7, 14
After the pain relief 6, 13

B
Back Pain Relief 8
Bed 6, 13
Body positioning 6
Breakfast 2, 9
Broccoli boiling time 14
Butter, margarine or cheese 3

D
Dental Pain Relief 1
Dinner 5, 12
Discovery of procedures for back pain relief iv
Discovery of procedures for dental pain relief iv
Discussion and Conclusion 7, 14
Duration of the boiling 12

E
Eating the breakfast 3, 10
Egg-tomato-onion combination 8
Exercising 5, 13
Extra broccoli benefit 14

F
Food Preparation Instructions 2, 9
Fruits 12

L
Lunch 4, 11

N
No alcohol 6, 13

P

Positive effects on the respiratory system. 14
Preparation of an Appetizing Ashanti Light Soup 4, 11
Proper positioning of the human body 1, 6

R

Reasons why sleeping on the 7

S

Seniors Walking With Canes 8
Sleeping on the stomach 6
Solution to Dental Pain Problems 1
Sunshine 6

W

Watching what you eat or drink 14
Water after every meal 3, 10

17

www.ingramcontent.com/pod-product-compliance
Lightning Source LLC
Chambersburg PA
CBHW081205020426
42333CB00020B/2628